A HANDBOOK OF AORTIC VALVE DISEASE

Alok Ranjan

MD, DNB, MRCP (UK), DM (Card.)
Sr. Consultant - Cardiology
Wockhardt Hospitals
India

authorHOUSE®

AuthorHouse™
1663 Liberty Drive
Bloomington, IN 47403
www.authorhouse.com
Phone: 1-800-839-8640

Published by AuthorHouse 3/13/2012

ISBN: 978-1-4685-4664-4 (e)
ISBN: 978-1-4685-4665-1 (hc)
ISBN: 978-1-4685-4666-8 (sc)

Library of Congress Control Number: 2012902172

Disclaimer

Medicine is a constantly changing science. New research findings necessitate continual changes in disease concept and its management. The author and publisher of this handbook have used reasonable efforts to provide up-to-date, accurate information that is within generally accepted medical standards at the time of publication. However, as medical science is ever evolving, and human error is always possible, the author and publisher (or any other involved parties) do not guarantee total accuracy or comprehensiveness of the information in this handbook, and they are not responsible for omissions, errors, or the results of using this information. The reader should confirm the accuracy of the information in this handbook from other sources. In particular, all drug doses, indications, and contraindications should be confirmed in package inserts.

The author has made every effort to trace the copyright holders for borrowed material. If he has inadvertently overlooked any, he will be pleased to make necessary arrangement at the first opportunity.

Dedicated to wife, Puja and kids, Adishree and Anirvan.

"Families are like fudge – mostly sweet with a few nuts"

Thank you for tolerating 'the nut'.

Contents

Aortic Stenosis

Introduction

Aortic stenosis is usually defined by restricted systolic opening of the valve leaflets, with a mean transvalvular pressure gradient of at least 5 - 10 mm Hg.

LVOTO (Left ventricular outflow tract obstruction) includes obstruction at valve, sub-valvular and supravalvular level.

The normal aortic valve is 3 to 4 sq. cm. in area when fully open.

The natural progression of Aortic Stenosis is slow and is from mild to moderate to severe stenosis. Development of symptoms indicates more than moderate Aortic Stenosis

Thus, AS is an insidious disease with a long latency period followed by rapid progression after the appearance of symptoms, resulting in a high rate of death (approximately 50% in the first 2 years after symptoms appear) among untreated patients.

Etiology

Causes of left ventricular outflow tract obstruction (LVOTO)

Valvular Aortic stenosis

Acquired
    Post inflammatory (usually rheumatic)
        The most distinctive aortic valve change secondary to valvulitis is commissural fusion, the single most important finding in determining that the cause is rheumatic (or post-inflammatory). Severe AS may be seen after brucellar or rickettsial infection.
    Degenerative
        Bi or tricuspid AV
            It is unusual for a bicuspid or tricuspid valve to be stenotic in absence of significant calcification. Non calcific AS with fibrosis is therefore more likely to be rheumatic in origin.
Congenital
        Unicuspid valve
        Tricuspid with fusion of commissures
        Hypoplastic annulus
Rare causes
        SLE (especially after steroid therapy)

Fabry's disease and Ochronosis (metabolic products accumulates in cusps)

Type II hyperlipoprotenemia

IE

Secondary to Radiotherapy

Nonvalvular aortic stenosis

Rare; as all acquired pathology and more than 70 % of congenital lesions are valvular stenosis

Subvalvular obstruction
        Discrete fibromembranous
        Diffuse fibromuscular (tunnel)
        Muscular (Hypertrophic subaortic stenosis)
Supravalvular obstruction
        Hourglass
        Hypoplastic
        Membranous

Age of presentation of LVOTO

Infancy to first decade:
        Congenital valvular, subvalvular or supravalvular pathology
Early childhood to late adulthood
        Rheumatic AS
        Hypertrophic subaortic stenosis
Early to late adulthood
        Degenerative AV disease
                Degenerative Tricuspid AV disease usually present after 65 yrs of age

Pathophysiology

Valvular aortic stenosis results in chronic left ventricular pressure over-loading. The AVA has to be reduced by about 50% of normal before a measurable gradient can be demonstrated in humans. Pure aortic valve stenosis results in compensatory ventricular hypertrophy proportional to the degree of obstruction. Mild degrees of obstruction are usually well tolerated, with minimal hypertrophy and normal left ventricular func-tion. As stenosis progresses, hypertrophy increases and reduces wall stress. In most patients with AS, cardiac output is in the normal range and initially increases normally with exercise. Eventually, however, left ventricular hypertrophy results in either 1) diastolic dysfunction with the onset of congestive symptoms, or 2) myocardial oxygen needs in excess of supply with the onset of angina. Some patients may also ex-perience exertional syncope, because as the severity of AS increases progressively, the cardiac output remains within the normal range at rest, but, on exercise, it no longer increases in proportion to the amount of exercise undertaken or does not increase at all (fixed cardiac output). With the development of heart failure, there is a reduction in the rest-ing cardiac output and tachycardia. As a result, stroke volume may be so lowered that it results in a small gradient across the left ventricular outflow tract in spite of severe AS.

At any stage of life, however, the natural history of aortic steno-sis largely reflects the functional integrity of the *mitral* valve. As long as adequate mitral valve function is maintained, the pulmonary bed is protected from the systolic pressure overloading imposed by aortic stenosis. In contrast to mitral valve disease where the pulmonary circuit is directly involved, compensatory concentric left ventricular hypertrophy allows the pressure overloaded ventricle to maintain stroke volume with modest increases in diastolic pressure, and patients can remain asymptomatic for many years.

Hemodynamics

Reduction in valve size more than 50 % results in increased gradient across AV.

For hemodynamically significant AS, valve area should be reduced by more than 60 %. At this stage compensatory mechanism in form of LV hypertrophy starts.

The hemodynamic characteristics of significant AS are:

Raised LVEDP

High 'a' wave in LA pressure trace

No increase in mean LAP, PAWP or RVSP in asymptomatic patients with normal LV function.

Unlike MS, the AV gradient does not increase with exercise because tachycardia mainly occurs at the expense of diastolic time.

Clinical features

Symptoms

Classical Triad

Angina
Syncope
Congestive Heart Failure

1. ANGINA (angina pectoris)

Presenting feature in 70 % cases;
Usually indicates severe AS; in only less than 10 % patients AS
    may not be severe.
Usually the initial symptom
More frequent with AS than any other valve lesions
Life expectancy less than 5 years after onset of angina
Typically exertional angina
    Mechanisms:
        Demand – supply mismatch
        Subendocardial ischemia
        Hypertrophied muscles more prone to ischemia
        Additional CAD

Responds to nitrate but avoid as nitrate induced hypotension can be dangerous

Angina at rest indicates associated coronary artery disease

2. SYNCOPE

Presenting feature in 33 % cases;

Indicates severe AS; only in less than 10% cases, AS may not be severe

Occurs during exercise as a consequence of
- Reduction of the systematic vascular resistance (Vasodilation in skeletal muscle)
- Failure of forearm vasoconstriction during leg exercise (Ventricular Bazold – Jarisch reflex)
- Failure of cardiac output to rise due to severe fixed obstruction
- Arrhythmias (Tachy or bradyarrhythmias): Can lead to syncope at rest also.

Syncope in 'mild AS': Causes
- Coronary artery disease
- Hypertrophic cardiomyopathy
- Unrelated non cardiac cause

3. CONGESTIVE HEART FAILURE (CHF)

Seen in 15 % cases

Symptoms include.
- Dyspnea.
- Orthopnea.
- Paroxysmal Noctural Dyspnea.
- Pulmonary Edema.
- Pulmonary Hypertension.
- End Stage: Right Ventricular Failure

Dyspnea in AS
Causes:
Diastolic dysfunction of LV
Congestive heart failure

Dyspnea in a case of 'Mild AS'
Associated Mitral valve disease; if in a case of RHD and AS, if the duration of dyspnea is **longer than 5 yrs**, then associated MV disease should be strongly suspected.
Hypertrophic cardiomyopathy
Coronary artery disease
Unrelated pathology (eg., Pulmonary cause)

Diastolic Dysfunction as cause of dyspnea:
It is a common cause of dyspnea on exertion in AS (seen in 45 % cases).
Mechanism:
AS leads to LV hypertrophy as a compensatory mechanism
Increase LV wall thickness reduces ventricular compliance:
Leads to raised LVEDP
The Atrium needs higher pressure to fill the ventricle:
Leads to raised LAP
Development of symptoms of pulmonary congestion due to raised LAP

This entity (diastolic dysfunction) **must be distinguished** from dyspnea due to CHF, which carries a grave prognosis.

Rare symptoms:

Systemic emboli
Usually silent

Due to
> Thrombus: Very rare
>> Hence long term anticoagulation is not indicated in AS
> Vegetation
> Calcium emboli

IE
> Risk of IE decreases as the extent of calcification increases
> Unrelated to severity of AS but is related to severity of AS in post AVR cases

GI bleeding: (mainly with degenerative AS): Hayde syndrome
> Rare
> The high shear stress of stenotic valves makes multi-meric Von Willebrand's factor more susceptible to cleavage by a plasma metalloprotease and may increase platelet clearance
> May also be due to arteriovenous malformations (angiodysplasia)
>> involving
>>> Right colon
>>> Small bowel
>>> Stomach
> Bleeding usually ceases with AVR

Signs

1. Pulse:
Always examine 'Carotid' pulse if AS is suspected
Classical finding:
> Pulsus parvus et tardus (Slow rising and small volume pulse)

More common in decompensated AS; usually associated with other signs of LV failure.

Other features:

Slow rising (pulsus parvus)

Delayed peak (pulsus tardus)

Reduced amplitude

Sustained contour

With or without thrill in 'carotid'

* A normal carotid pulse in an adult with clinically normal LV function excludes moderate to severe AS.

Factors that 'mask' the typical quality of AS pulse

Associated AR

Associated systemic hypertension

High cardiac output states

Young patients (elastic arterial walls)

Elderly patients (arteriosclerosis)

CCF

Atrial Fibrillation: Always rule out co-existent MV disease

Symptoms may appear as atrial contraction contributes up to 40 % of the ventricular filling during diastole in AS (atrial contraction contributes nearly 20 % in a normal heart)

AF may cause rapid deterioration of clinical features of AS

2. Blood pressure:

Normal in most cases

Abnormal if associated with systemic hypertension or with associated AR.

May have narrow pulse pressure in severe AS (not a rule)

High systolic BP does not rule out significant AS unless more than 250 mm Hg

3. Apical impulse

LV type

Heaving in character,

At normal site (5th ICS, inside mid clavicular line: suggestive of absence of cardiomegaly)

Cardiomegaly in case of pure AS indicates CHF and grave prognosis.

Palpable S4

    Usually indicates AV gradient more than 70 mm Hg

    May be present even if S4 is not 'audible'

4. Systolic thrill

Is a rule if **significant** AS is present.

Most commonly felt in 'aortic' area; radiates to neck, right supraclavicular or shoulder

Does not always indicate 'severe' AS

5. Jugular Venous Pulse in AS

Feature	Findings	Mechanism / significance
Level	Normal or elevated	Elevated with RV failure secondary to LV failure Associated MS with PAH Associated organic TS
Waves		
A	Normal or prominent	**Prominent A wave with** Severe AS; Severe IVS hypertrophy leads to reduced RV compliance If associated with MS and PH / TS HOCM

| V/X/Y; | Normal | Abnormal with RV failure or TV disease |

6. Auscultation
Ascultation: Sounds

- S1: Normal and unremarkable
  Loud S1
  > Associated MS
  > Think of Aortic EC !!
  >> A 'loud and discrete' S1 at aortic or pulmonary area is usually EC rather than S1 in a case suspected to be of AS
  Soft S1:
  > LV dysfunction
  > Raised LVEDP
- S2:
  Intensity: A2: Soft; P2: Normal
  Soft A2
  > Indicates fibrotic and calcific valve
  > Usual in rheumatic or degenerative AS
  > Hence, **Classically, A2 is diminished to absent** (seen in 20% cases);
  Normal A2: Rare; seen in 10 % cases; According to Paul Wood, normal A2 is present only in 5% cases of acquired AS
  Normal or increased A2
  > *Indicates pliable and relatively thin leaflet
  > Usual in 'Congenital' AS

  Splitting of S2
  > Normal split: Rules out significant AS. Seen in
  >> Mild AS
  >> Congenital AS

*Hemodynamically significant AS has abnormal splitting of S2

Single S2 (seen in 70 % cases)
   Due to A2 'moving into' P2
   Can also be due to 'soft' A2 because of fibrocalfic valve
       Decreased intensity of A2 and hence only P2 is heard
Reverse split of S2 (seen in 20% cases);
   Always indicates severe AS;
   Reverse A2 P2 split does **not** indicate severe AS if associated with AR.

- S3: Never heard except in CHF (late stage of AS) and in young patient.

- S4: Always present.
      A palpable S4 indicates severe AS; although unreliable sign of severe AS if patient is more than 45 yrs of age
      Palpable S4 indicates an LVEDP > 15 mm Hg.
      Palpable S4 rules out associated MS
- Aortic EC:
      Intensity of EC mirrors that of A2
      It confirms the diagnosis of structural heart disease in a case of ejection systolic murmur
      Localizes the disease to valve; in absence of dilated aorta or chronic hypertension
      Usually it is due to 'congenital' deformity of valve; almost a rule in congenital AS but present in less than 1/3rd patients with AS with more than 50 yrs of age
      Uncommon in tricuspid AV with acquired stenosis
      More common in less severe AS

Mild to moderate AS (75%) & severe AS (25 %)

Hence presence of EC does not predict severity of AS

*A 'loud and discrete' S1 at aortic or pulmonary area is usually EC rather than S1 in a case suspected to be of AS

Auscultation: Murmur

- ESM

    Best heard in 'aortic' area

    Radiates to carotids and to apex (Gallavardin phenomenon)

    Late peaking murmur indicates severe AS

    More reliable than length of murmur in assessing severity

    Length of murmur is proportional to severity of AS in absence of AR and LVF

    Thrill (seen in 80% cases):

    Thrill does not indicate severe AS; loudness does NOT correlate with severity.

    Loudness does not correlate severity except in congenital AS (Ref.: Abrams)

    * Characteristics of murmur do not differentiate congenital vs. acquired or valvular vs. either sub or supravalvular AS

Criteria for Severe AS

Symptomatic patient

Low volume & slow rising pulse with decreased carotid pulsation

Palpable S4

Paradoxical A2 – P2 split

Long and late peaking ESM with absent EC

Criteria for CRITICAL AS

- Valve Area <0.7cm2
- Increase LVEDP
- Decreased LVEF
- Decreased Stroke Volume

Investigations

1. ECG

Almost always abnormal (except in 10 % cases) if AS is severe.

In pure AS, the total 12 lead QRS amplitude in millimeters is equal
to LV systolic pressure in mm Hg.

More reliable in congenital AS

Presence of Left ventricular hypertrophy (LVH)

Presence of left atrial enlargement (LAE):

Should raise suspicion of coexisting MV disease but LAE may
be present in severe AS without MV disease

LAE is present in > 80 % cases with severe isolated AS

Conduction blocks:

More common in AS than any other valve lesions: 5 % cases

Bundle Branch Block

1st degree heart block

Complete Heart Block

Due to

Septal trauma due to high intra-myocardial
tension

Hypoxic damage to conducting fibers

Extension of valvular calcification

AF:

Seen in only 10 – 15 % cases

Its presence should raise a suspicion of coexisting MVD

2. CXR

Normal Heart size with increased convexity of the left ventricular silhouette due to ventricular hypertrophy

Calcification of the Aortic Valve:

Usually with valvular AS

Better seen on fluoroscopy and in lateral or oblique views on CXR

Absence of calcification in a patient more than 40 yrs. (not valid for younger patients) rules out significant AS.

Absence of calcification can **not** be concluded on CXR only.

Fluoroscopy or CT scan are more diagnostic

Ascending aorta dilation: Present;

Usually only with valvular AS (seen in 80 % cases)

Absent in nonvalvular stenosis or coexisting mitral valve disease

Magnitude of dilation does not correlate with severity

Cardiomegaly in end stage disease

* A normal CXR does not rule out severe AS

3. Stress Test

Role of Treadmill stress testing

Dangerous in symptomatic patients

Not useful for diagnosis of CAD

May be used to assess functional significance of severe AS in patients who deny symptoms (e.g., hypotensive response to exercise)

4. ECHOCARDIOGRAPHY

Very useful in diagnosis and management of AS.

Confirms diagnosis of AS and its severity

Defines etiology of AS

Differentiates valvular with non valvular AS

Points to remember in echocardiographic evaluation of AS

Motility of the Leaflet; calcification of valve

Gradient across the valve

Measurement of the valve areas

LVEF

Regional Ventricular Motion

Ventricular Hypertrophy

Left Atrial Enlargement

To rule out other congenital heart disease (specially in children)

AS: M Mode features

Dimensions of cardiac chambers

Severity of LVH

Closure line of AV

Thick and central: Tricuspid AV

Thick and eccentric: Bicuspid AV

Reduced separation of AV leaflets

Normal 16 to 21 mm

Reduced < 10 mm

D/D with HOCM: Points favoring HOCM

Asymmetrical septal hypertrophy

SAM of AML

Bicuspid Aortic Valve
M-Mode

Thickened aortic valve leaflets

Eccentric closure line of aortic valve leaflets. The degree of eccentricity can be calculated as:

$$EI = 1/2 \, A \div a$$

Where EI is the eccentricity index, A is the internal aortic root diameter at the onset of diastole, and a is the distance from the line of aortic cusp coaptation to the nearest aortic wall at the onset of diastole.

An index ≥ 1.5 indicates a bicuspid aortic valve (74% of patients who have surgically or angiographically proved bicuspid aortic valve). A normal eccentricity index (< 1. 5) does not exclude the presence of a bicuspid aortic valve.

AS: 2 – D Echo features

Rules out coexisting valve disease
Morphology of AV: number of cusps
Mobility of leaflets
Calcification of leaflets: Important for advising against BAV

PLAX:
    Leaflets seen in this view are right coronary cusp (anterior cusp) and non coronary cusp (posterior)
    Measurement of aortic annulus and ascending aorta
    Thickness, doming and calcification of valve
    Vegetation
    To rule out sub or supravalvular AS
PSAX:
    Morphology of AV leaflets (number, thickness, calcification etc)
    AV Area measurement
        Use end systolic planimetery area
        TEE is superior to TTE for area measurement
    LVEF
Apical views:
    LVEF
    Site of obstruction (Valve / LVOT or supravalvular)
Color Doppler

Gradient across AV (AVG)
Best in A4C view
Other views
Suprasternal
Right parasternal

AS: Grading of severity

Grade	AVA (sq. cm)	Peak AVG (mm Hg)	Mean AVG (mm Hg)
Mild	> 1.5 (> 0.9 cm^2/m^2)	< 40	< 25
Moderate	1.0 – 1.5 (0.6-0.9 cm^2/m^2)	40 – 70	25 - 40
Severe	≤ 1.0 (< 0.6 cm^2/m^2)	> 70	> 40

AS: Measurement of AV area on Echocardiography

Continuity equation
Planimetery

Continuity Equation:

$$AVA = \text{Area LVOT} \times VTI_{LVOT} / VTI_{AV}$$
$$= D^2 \times 0.785 \times VTI_{LVOT} / VTI_{AV}$$

For clinical use maximal velocity can be substituted for VTI

$$AVA = \text{Area LVOT} \times V_{LVOT} / V_{AV}$$
$$= D^2 \times 0.785 \times V_{LVOT} / V_{AV}$$

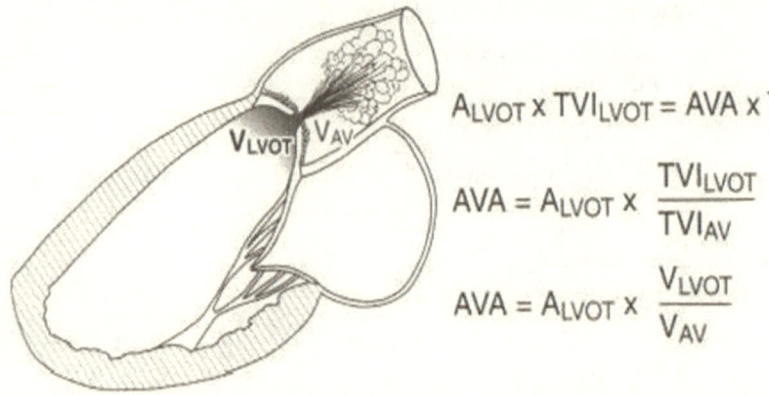

$$A_{LVOT} \times TVI_{LVOT} = AVA \times TVI_{AV}$$

$$AVA = A_{LVOT} \times \frac{TVI_{LVOT}}{TVI_{AV}}$$

$$AVA = A_{LVOT} \times \frac{V_{LVOT}}{V_{AV}}$$

Where D is LVOT diameter measured in PLAX in mid systole

VTI_{LVOT} measured by PW Doppler placed proximal to AV

VTI_{AV} measured by CW Doppler of AV velocity

V_{LVOT} is maximum velocity measured by PW Doppler positioned 3-5 mm below AV

V_{AV} is maximum velocity measured by CW Doppler of AV velocity

Planimetery

Best by TEE

Flow Velocity Ratio

Indexed valve area for body size

If "Normal" AVA = CSA $_{LVOT}$ and,

Actual AVA x V_{AO} = "Normal" AVA x V_{LVOT},

then, Actual AVA / "Normal" AVA = V_{LVOT}/V_{AO}

V_{LVOT}/V_{AO} less than 0.25 signifies severe aortic stenosis

Where

CSA $_{LVOT}$: Cross sectional area of LVOT

V_{LVOT} is maximum velocity measured by PW Doppler

positioned 3 – 5 mm below AV

V_{AV} is maximum velocity measured by CW Doppler of AV velocity

Special clinical situation of low AV gradient with LV dysfunction

Low flow and low gradient AS: Defined as
  AVA < 1.0 sq. cm
  LVEF < 40 %
  Mean AVG < 30-40 mm Hg

Low AV gradient in presence of LV systolic dysfunction poses a diagnostic dilemma. It is important to ascertain whether the low AV gradient is due to poor LV function or the severity of AS is of milder degree.

D/D Dilated Cardiomyopathy with calcific AV that is not stenotic

Criteria of severe AS in presence of poor LV function:

AVA < 0.25 cm^2 (The cut off value with good LV function is < 0.75 cm^2)

Ratio of VTI $_{LVOT}$ / VTI $_{AV}$ is less than 0.25

Dobutamine Stress Echo
  Doses: Up to 20 mcg / kg / min
  True severe AS:
    AV gradient increases
    Velocity increases to at least 4 m / sec
    Ratio of VTI $_{LVOT}$ / VTI $_{AV}$ is less than 0.25
  Pseudo severe AS
    AS gradient does not increase

Ratio of VTI $_{LVOT}$ / VTI $_{AV}$ is more than 0.25

VTI $_{LVOT}$ increases as area is higher with high output

Summary of Criteria of Severe AS on echocardiography

Peak AV gradient > 70 mm Hg or peak velocity > 4.5 m / sec

Mean AV gradient > 40 mm Hg

AVA is < 0.75 cm²

Ratio of VTI $_{LVOT}$ / VTI $_{AV}$ is less than 0.25

Aortic Valve resistance (Bermejo et al; JACC 1996; 26; 1206-13)

> Good correlation with aortic valve area for a given aortic flow velocity
>
> Less affected by a change in flow
>
> Not better than other measurements

Mean resistance = 28 x Mean AVG / AVA

4. AS: ANGIOGRAM

Echo measurements are accurate to diagnose severe AS. However AV gradient at Echo-Doppler study usually overestimates the gradient because instantaneous gradient rather than peak to peak gradient is measured in Echo. However, several studies have confirmed that the Doppler derived pressure gradients across AV and AVA correlates well with catheter derived pressure gradient.

Cardiac Catheterization

- Determines peak-to-peak pressure gradient
- Determines mean pressure gradient
- Determines aortic valve area by the Gorlin formula:
  AVA (cm2) = (CO ÷ SEP) ÷ (43. 3 x MPG)
  Where AVA is the aortic valve area, CO is cardiac output, SEP

the systolic ejection period, 43.3 is the constant, and MPG is the mean pressure gradient

- Catheterization study mainly indicated in patients over 35 yrs to exclude coexisting CAD
- Also identifies Coronary Anomalies: LCX dominant circulation is more common
- Aortogram to identify post stenotic dilation
- Calcium deposits in the Aortic wall

Natural History

Salient points:
- Long asymptomatic period
- When symptoms develop, duration of life is markedly reduced
- After angina occurs, survival is approximately 4yrs. After onset of syncope the survival period is approximately 2yrs and is less than 1 yr after onset of congestive heart failure (Worse than the 5, 3 and 2 yrs reported by Ross and Braunwald from 7 autopsy series)
- Valve area is not the only prognostic factor
- Absence of symptoms does not guarantee absence of LV dysfunction
- Sudden cardiac death is seen in more than 10% in **symptomatic** patients; SCD is not common in asymptomatic patient with severe AS and normal LV function.

Natural History of symptomatic severe AS

- Ross & Braunwald: Analysis of 7 autopsy studies before 1955
  - Average life expectancy: 3 yrs
    - After onset of Angina: 5 yrs
    - After onset of Syncope: 3 yrs
    - After onset of CHF: 2 yrs

  Sudden Death: Responsible for 15 – 20 % of total deaths. 65 – 80 % of sudden deaths occurred in symptomatic patients.

- Horstkotte and Loogan

  N = 35

  AVA: < 0.8 sq. cm

  Consisted of a group of patients who refused surgery and were symptomatic

  5 yr mortality rate was 82 +/- 7 %

  All patients died within 12 yrs.

  Conclusion: The average survival after onset of symptoms was 23 months; the mean survival after occurrence of angina was 45 months, after syncope was 27 months and after onset of left heart failure was 11 months.

- Rapaport:

  Mortality rate

At 5 yrs:	60 %
At 10 yrs:	80 %

  Summary: Symptomatic AS is associated with a high or very high mortality rate when managed medically; the mortality rate is much higher than that of many malignant neoplasms.

Natural History of asymptomatic severe AS:

Limited studies are available.
- Kelly et al:

  N = 51;

  Follow up period: 17 ± 9 months;

  Symptoms developed in 4 patients and 16 patients died (Total: 20; 57%);

  However only 2 died of SCD (sudden cardiac death)

- Ross & Braunwald: concluded that 3-5 % of deaths in acquired AS occurred suddenly in asymptomatic patients.

- Horskotte & Loogen : 3 out of 10 patients (30 %) died before onset of symptoms

- Tajik:
  N = 143;
  30 required AVR; 113 did not require AVR;
  But 3 died; all became symptomatic before death

Natural History of moderate AS

- Horskotte and Loogan:
  Defined moderate AS as AVA 0.8 – 1.5 sq. cm and AV gradient as $\leq$ 80 mm Hg.
  In this group of patients, at 10 yrs of follow up, deterioration was seen in 30 % cases. It progressed to severe AS in 5 % cases and in another 25 % cases, AVR was performed.

  However this group can not be considered to comprise the real moderate AS cases only, due to their definition of moderate AS.
  Hence the study does not truly reflect natural history of moderate AS.

- Another study:
  N=66;
  AVA: 0.7 – 1.2 sq. cm.
  Follow up period: 35 months;
    14 patients died
    25 patients required AVR;
  The estimated probability of remaining free of any complications of AS at the end of 4 yrs is 59 %
  This study also had a mixed population of moderate and severe AS.

Natural History of mild AS:

Horskotte & Loogan;
   N = 142

AVA > 1.5 sq.cm.

Follow up period: More than 25 yrs.

Grade	Survival Rate and severity of AS		
	At 10 yr (%)	At 20 yr (%)	At 25 yr (%)
Mild	88	63	38
Moderate	4	15	25
Severe AS / AVR	8	22	38

Conclusion: Patients with aortic valve area > 1.5 sq. cm (mild AS) should not undergo valve surgery or other intervention therapy.

Rate of progression of AS (based on these studies)
   AVA decrease by 0.1 – 0.5 cm^2 per year
   Mean pressure gradient increase by 7 – 23 mm Hg per year
   Increase in velocity is 0.3 – 1.0 m /sec per year

   According to Braunwald's Text book:
      Annual decrease in AVA of 0.12 sq. cm. / yr
      Increase in aortic jet velocity of 0.32 m/sec/year
      Increase in mean AVG of 7 mm Hg/year
      However, the rate of progression is variable and rapid in older age, more severe valve calcification, renal insufficiency, hypertension, smoking and hyperlipidemia.

Management

Options:

1. Medical treatment: Limited role
2. Interventions

AS: Medical Therapy

Indicated only as pre-operative management in severe symptomatic AS awaiting surgery.

Diuretics for heart failure

ACE inhibitors in carefully selected cases of heart failure

Beta Blockers for Angina

No proven preventive treatment: Recent report suggest use of lipid lowering therapy (Statins) may slow the progression of calcific Aortic Stenosis

Patient education about AS and its natural history so that interventions can be performed as soon as symptoms develop, is very important

Medical therapy: Useful in inoperable cases of AS

AS: Interventions

Options:
Transcatheter
Balloon Aortic Valvotomy
> For congenital AS

Transcatheter aortic-valve implantation (TAVI)
> For seriously ill patients who are not candidate for conventional surgery

Surgery
Aortic Valve replacement
> Either with metallic or bioprosthetic valve

Open Aortic Valvotomy
> Simple commissural incision under direct vision
> For congenital AS

Ross procedure

Interventions: Indications

Symptomatic Severe AS:
> Reason: Improves survival after surgery
> 5 yrs: Survival rate is 75 – 80 %
> 10 yrs.   Survival rate is 60 %

Asymptomatic Severe AS: Indicated in children only; as BAV is feasible and is associated with very low mortality

Asymptomatic severe AS with high risk of SCD (> 3 –5 %)
- Evidence of progressive LV dysfunction
- Significant ventricular ectopy
- Abnormal hemodynamic response to TMT

Do not intervene if

Asymptomatic Severe AS: Because the operative mortality

is more than the incidence of SCD and hence surgery is not advised. In children BAV is the treatment of choice and the operative risk is < 1 %. Hence in children severe asymptomatic AS should be intervened (with BAV).

Moderate AS:

Do not operate;

No definite guidelines if associated with multivalvular disease;

Do not operate in CABG (Avoid concomitant AVR if AS is moderate in severity at the time of CABG)

Low Gradient AS

Special case

Minimal valve mobility and low cardiac output

Calculated valve area is small but pressure gradient is also small

Dilemma between Functional vs. fixed AS

Consider dobutamine stress test (DSE) to clarify

AVR should be considered if the mean AVG is > 20 mm Hg because survival after AVR is better (~ 50 % at 5 yrs) than medical therapy.

Indications for Aortic Valve Replacement

Class I

1. AVR is indicated for symptomatic patients with severe AS.* *(Level of Evidence: B)*
2. AVR is indicated for patients with severe AS* undergoing coronary artery bypass graft surgery (CABG). *(Level of Evidence: C)*
3. AVR is indicated for patients with severe AS* undergoing surgery on the aorta or other heart valves. *(Level of Evidence: C)*

4. AVR is recommended for patients with severe AS* and LV systolic dysfunction (ejection fraction less than 0.50). *(Level of Evidence: C)*

Class IIa

AVR is reasonable for patients with moderate AS* undergoing CABG or surgery on the aorta or other heart valves *(Level of Evidence: B)*

Class IIb

1. AVR may be considered for asymptomatic patients with severe AS* and abnormal response to exercise (e.g., development of symptoms or asymptomatic hypotension). *(Level of Evidence: C)*
2. AVR may be considered for adults with severe asymptomatic AS* if there is a high likelihood of rapid progression (age, calcification, and CAD) or if surgery might be delayed at the time of symptom onset. *(Level of Evidence: C)*
3. AVR may be considered in patients undergoing CABG who have mild AS* when there is evidence, such as moderate to severe valve calcification, that progression may be rapid. *(Level of Evidence: C)*
4. AVR may be considered for asymptomatic patients with extremely severe AS (aortic valve area less than 0.6 cm², mean gradient greater than 60 mm Hg, and jet velocity greater than 5.0 m per second) when the patient's expected operative mortality is 1.0% or less. *(Level of Evidence: C)*

Class III

AVR is not useful for the prevention of sudden death in asymptomatic patients with AS who have none of the findings listed under the class IIa/IIb recommendations. *(Level of Evidence: B)*
*: Grading of severity of AS as defined on page 25

Aortic Valve Replacement in Patients Undergoing Coronary Artery Bypass Surgery

Class I

AVR is indicated in patients undergoing CABG who have severe AS who meet the criteria for valve replacement (see Section 3.1.7 of the original guideline document). *(Level of Evidence: C)*

Class IIa

AVR is reasonable in patients undergoing CABG who have moderate AS (mean gradient 30 to 50 mm Hg or Doppler velocity 3 to 4 m per second). *(Level of Evidence: B)*

Class IIb

AVR may be considered in patients undergoing CABG who have mild AS (mean gradient less than 30 mm Hg or Doppler velocity less than 3 m per second) when there is evidence, such as moderate-severe valve calcification, that progression may be rapid. *(Level of Evidence: C)*

Major Criteria for Aortic Valve Selection

Class I

1. A mechanical prosthesis is recommended for AVR in patients with a mechanical valve in the mitral or tricuspid position. *(Level of Evidence: C)*
2. A bioprosthesis is recommended for AVR in patients of any age who will not take warfarin or who have major medical contraindications to warfarin therapy. *(Level of Evidence: C)*

Class IIa

1. Patient preference is a reasonable consideration in the selection of aortic valve operation and valve prosthesis. A mechanical prosthesis is reasonable for AVR in patients under 65 years of age who do not have a contraindication to anticoagulation. A bioprosthesis is reasonable for AVR in patients under 65 years of age who elect to receive this valve for lifestyle considerations after detailed discussions of the risks of anticoagulation versus the likelihood that a second AVR may be necessary in the future. *(Level of Evidence: C)*
2. A bioprosthesis is reasonable for AVR in patients aged 65 years or older without risk factors for thromboembolism. *(Level of Evidence: C)*
3. Aortic valve re-replacement with a homograft is reasonable for patients with active prosthetic valve endocarditis. *(Level of Evidence: C)*

Class IIb

A bioprosthesis might be considered for AVR in a woman of childbearing age. *(Level of Evidence: C)*

Interventions in AS

1. AVR
- 1st performed in 1960
- Operative mortality: 3 –5 %
- Increased mortality with
  Emergency AVR
  Higher NYHA class ($\geq$ 3)
  Age > 65 yrs
  Critical AS : AVA < 0.7; LVEDP > 20 mm Hg
  LV dysfunction
  Presence of atrial fibrillation

Redo procedure

Concomitant CABG

- Factors affecting long term survival:

    Pre operative NYHA class

    Use of mechanical valve

    Age > 65 yrs

    Pre operative ventricular arrhythmias

    Post operative Bundle Branch Block

    LV dysfunction

    - Systolic dysfunction
    - Diastolic dysfunction: if LAP > 15 mmHg
      PAP > 24 mm Hg

However, in clinical practice, at least 30% of patients with severe symptomatic aortic stenosis do not undergo surgery for replacement of the aortic valve, owing to advanced age, left ventricular dysfunction, or the presence of multiple coexisting conditions. For these patients, option of Trans-catheter aortic valve implantation (TAVI) is now available.

Society of Thoracic Surgeons (STS) and logistic Euroscore are currently used to as a main inclusion criteria to identify high risk or inoperable patients for trans-catheter aortic valve implantation (TAVI). STS score is superior to the logistic Euroscore in predicting mortality in high risk patients with severe AS. These scores can be calculated online on their respective website addresses..

High surgical risk:

    STS score >10% or

    Logistic EuroSCORE >20%

2. Balloon Aortic Valvotomy (BAV)

- The increase in AVA after BAV is 0.3 – 0.4 sq. cm only

- Restenosis rate is high and occurs rapidly: 65 - 77 % cases show restenosis at 6 months and rate is higher if AVA after BAV is < 0.7 sq. cm

- High complication rate:
  Cummulative rate: 25 %;
  Procedure mortality: 3 –5 %
  In Hospital mortality: 7 –13 %
  Mortality at 6 months: 15 –22 %

Aortic Balloon Valvotomy: Indications

Class IIb

1. Aortic balloon valvotomy might be reasonable as a bridge to surgery in hemodynamically unstable adult patients with AS who are at high risk for AVR. *(Level of Evidence: C)*
2. Aortic balloon valvotomy might be reasonable for palliation in adult patients with AS in whom AVR cannot be performed because of serious comorbid conditions. *(Level of Evidence: C)*

Class III

Aortic balloon valvotomy is not recommended as an alternative to AVR in adult patients with AS; certain younger adults without valve calcification may be an exception *(Level of Evidence: B)*

BAV: Indications (Rahimtoola ; JACC 1989; vol 14(1): 1-23)
- High risk for cardiac surgery (CHF/LV dysfunction)
- Limited life span
- Urgent need for non cardiac surgical procedures
- Cardiac surgery undesirable for non cardiac reasons
- Patient with CHF of uncertain origin and AS of uncertain severity
- Refusal of Surgery

BAV for Congenital AS

Treatment of choice in congenital AS

Nonsurgical procedure in which a balloon-tipped catheter is passed through the narrowed aortic valve and inflated

Approach:

Retrograde: Femoral / Carotid / Scapular / Umbilical artery

Antegrade: Through atrial septum

- Lock JE et al; JACC 1996

    N=148; Age: > 1 month

    Success rate: 87%;

    Procedure mortality: 0.7%

    F/U: 6 yrs;

    Survival: 95 %

    Frequency of repeat intervention:

    50 % at 8yr follow up

    75% of these 80 % within 4yr

    Factors that increase risk of repeat intervention

    - Symmetrically thin or thick valves
    - High residual gradient
    - Post BAV; Severity of AR $\geq$ 3/4 grade

Lock JE: BAV in adults for congenital AS

    N = 18

    Age : 17 – 40 yrs

    Suboptimal result in 2 patients (required AVR)

    Death: 0

    F/U: 1 – 82 months

    - 8 patients: Symptom free
    - 3 patients: Required AVR

- VACA registry

    N = 630

Median age: 6.8 yrs (1 day – 18 yrs)
Procedure could not be performed: 4.1 %
Procedure related mortality: 1.9 %
Size of balloon: 0.9 – 1.0 times aortic root annulus
(Valve diameter)
Suboptimal result: 17 %;
Reasons
Failure to perform BAV
Residual gradient > 60 mm Hg
LV / Aorta pressure ≥ 1.6
Major complication / death

- BAV after Surgical valvotomy

N = 22
Mean F/U: 33 months
7/22 required reinterventions

Conclusion: Safe, feasible but high restenosis rate

3. Transcatheter aortic-valve implantation (TAVI)

Catheter-based aortic valve implantation
Has shown promising results in providing treatment options
for patients with severe AS who are poor open surgical
candidates
First performed: 2002: Alen Cribier et al.
3 catheter-based bioprosthetic aortic valves have been used in
human trials:
1. Cribier-Edwards valve (Edwards Lifesciences
Corporation, Irvine, CA),
2. Medtronic CoreValve (Medtronic Inc, Minneapolis,
Minnesota), and
3. The Edwards Sapien valve (Edwards Lifesciences
Corporation, Irvine, CA).

They have been implanted in humans utilizing three basic approaches:

1) transapical placement through a direct apical puncture;
2) retrograde transfemoral approach through the femoral artery, and;
3) antegrade transfemoral approach through the femoral vein.

   Transaxillary and transcarotid approaches have also been utilized successfully

Society of Thoracic Surgeons (STS) and logistic Euroscore are currently used as a main inclusion criteria to identify high risk or inoperable patients for trans-catheter aortic valve implantation (TAVI).

Basic procedural steps:

1. A standard BAV is performed
2. Transfemoral insertion of either a 22 or 24 Fr sheath, depending on the selected size of valve
3. The bioprosthetic heart valve, crimped onto a balloon catheter, is advanced across the native aortic valve. During rapid right ventricular pacing, balloon inflation of the crimped heart valve and support frame will simultaneously deploy the bioprosthetic valve and expanded the frame, which is secured to the underlying aortic-valve annulus and leaflets

Table: Differences between the Medtronic CoreValve and Edwards Sapien valve systems

	Medtronic CoreValve	Edwards Sapien valve
Minimum femoral artery diameter required	6.5 mm	7 mm
Composition	Porcine pericardial with nitinol stent	Bovine pericardial with steel stent
Delivery system size required	18 French	18 French (Sapien XT only)* 22 French (23 mm valve) 24 French (26 mm valve)
Native annulus size feasible for implant	19 mm to 27 mm	17 mm to 25 mm
Mechanism of implantation	Self-expanding	Balloon expandable
Ventricular rhythm at time of implant	Beating heart	Rapid ventricular pacing

* Currently not available in the U.S.

Bacterial Endocarditis in AS
- Staphylococcus aureus is the most common organism
- Infection most commonly causes valvular incompetence (regurgitation) from destruction of the valve and supporting structures
- Virulent cases can be seen in IV drug abusers who use unsterile needles

Aortic Regurgitation

Introduction

Aortic regurgitation (AR), also known as aortic insufficiency (AI), is incompetency of the aortic valve causing flow from the aorta into the left ventricle during diastole.

In individuals with a normally functioning aortic valve, the valve opens when the pressure in the left ventricle is higher than the pressure in the aorta. This allows the blood to be ejected from the left ventricle into the aorta during ventricular systole (Stroke volume). After ventricular systole, the pressure in the left ventricle decreases as it relaxes and begins to fill up with blood from the left atrium. This relaxation of the left ventricle (early ventricular diastole) causes a fall in its pressure. When the pressure in the left ventricle falls below the pressure in the aorta, the aortic valve will close, preventing blood in the aorta from going back into the left ventricle.

In AR, when the pressure in the left ventricle falls below the pressure in the aorta, the aortic valve is not able to close completely. This leads to leaking of blood from the aorta into the left ventricle. The percentage of blood that regurgitates back through the aortic valve due to AR is known as the regurgitant fraction.

Etiology

Chronic Aortic Regurgitation

Leaflet involvement

    RHD
    Congenital
        Unicuspid, bicuspid or quadricuspid valve
        Myxomatous degeneration
        Aneurysm of sinus of Valsalva
    Infective endocarditis

Aortic root dilatation

    Systemic Hypertension: Most common cause of mild AR
    Aortoarteritis
    Syphilis
    SLE
    Rheumatoid arthritis
    Ankylosing spondylitis
    Reiter's syndrome
    Heritable disorders of connective tissue disorders
    Marfan's syndrome
    Ehlers-Danlos syndrome

Pseudoxanthoma elasticum
Osteogenesis imperfecta

Loss of support

VSD

Abnormal channels

Aortic LV tunnel

Acute Aortic Regurgitation

Leaflet involvement

Infective endocarditis
Trauma

Aortic root dilatation

Aortic dissection

Abnormal channels

RSOV

Pathophysiology

In AR, since some of the blood that is ejected during systole regurgitates back into the left ventricle during diastole, *there is decreased effective forward flow.*

While diastolic blood pressure is diminished and the pulse pressure widens, systolic blood pressure generally remains normal or can even be slightly elevated. This is because sympathetic nervous system and the renin-angiotensin-aldosterone axis of the kidneys compensate for the decreased cardiac output. Catecholamines will increase the heart rate and increase the strength of ventricular contraction, directly increasing cardiac output. Catecholamines will also cause peripheral vasoconstriction, which causes increased systemic vascular resistance and ensures that core organs are adequately perfused. Renin, a proteolytic enzyme, cleaves angiotensinogen to angiotensin I, which is converted to angiotensin II, which is also a potent vasoconstrictor. In the case of chronic aortic insufficiency with resultant cardiac remodeling, heart failure will develop, and it is possible to see systolic pressures diminish.

Aortic insufficiency causes both volume overload (elevated preload) and pressure overload (elevated afterload) of the heart. The pressure overload (due to elevated pulse pressure and the systemic effects of neuroendocrine hormones) causes left ventricular hypertrophy (LVH). There is both **concentric hypertrophy** and **eccentric hypertrophy** in AR. The concentric hypertrophy is due to the increased left ventricular systolic pressures associated with AR, while the eccentric hypertrophy is due to volume overload caused by the regurgitant fraction. Mitral regurgitation constitutes a nearly pure volume overload wherein the excess volume is ejected against relatively low pressure into the left atrium. On the other hand, aortic regurgitation represents a combined pressure and volume overload in which the excess volume being pumped is ejected against the relatively high pressure of the aorta.

As the severity of AR increases, larger volume of blood regurgitates into left ventricle in each diastole. A series of compensatory mechanisms (Increased End Diastolic Volumes, Increased chamber compliance, combined eccentric and concentric hypertrophy) are produced by the LV to handle the volume overload. A majority of patients remain asymptomatic during this compensated phase. The transition to LV systolic dysfunction represents a continuum. Initially it is because of afterload mismatch and later due to intrinsic depression in contractility. LV systolic function and end systolic size have been identified as important determinants of survival and post operative LV function in patients undergoing AVR for chronic AR

Hemodynamics

The hemodynamic sequelae of AR are dependent on the rate of onset of AR. Acute AR and chronic AR will have different hemodynamics and individuals will have different signs and symptoms.

Acute aortic regurgitation

In acute AR, there will be a sudden increase in the volume of blood in the left ventricle. The ventricle is unable to deal with the sudden change in volume. In terms of the Frank-Starling curve, the end-diastolic volume will be very high, such that further increases in volume result in less and less efficient contraction. The filling pressure of the left ventricle will increase. This causes pressure in the left atrium to rise, and the individual will develop pulmonary edema.

Acute AR usually presents as florid congestive heart failure, and will not have any of the signs associated with chronic AR since the left ventricle has not yet developed the eccentric hypertrophy and dilatation that allow an increased stroke volume, which in turn causes bounding peripheral pulses.

Acute AR:

Very high LVEDP

Raised 'a' wave in LV pressure trace

Chronic aortic regurgitation

The left ventricle adapts by eccentric hypertrophy and dilatation of the left ventricle, and the volume overload is compensated for. The left ventricular filling pressures will revert to normal and the individual will no longer have overt heart failure.

In this compensated phase, the individual may be totally asymptomatic and may have normal exercise tolerance.

Eventually (typically after a latency period) the left ventricle will become decompensated, and filling pressures will increase. While most individuals would complain of symptoms of congestive heart failure to their physicians, some enter this decompensated phase asymptomatically. Proper treatment for AI involves aortic valve replacement prior to this decompensation phase.

Chronic AR

    LVEDP: Mildly increased in hemodynamically compensated AR

    Chronic severe AR

        Mild to moderate decompensation:

            Raised LVEDP

            High LAP

            High PAWP

        Severe decompensation

            All of the above and

            Raised RAP

            Raised RVEDP

    Cardiac output: Normal in compensated state

    LA / RA size: Normal in compensated state

    RV: Normal in compensated state

    PAWP: Normal in compensated state

Chronic AR: Clinical Features

May remain asymptomatic for decades

Symptoms

Dyspnea
    Dyspnea especially on exertion or on lying flat
    Orthopnea and PND after onset of LV dysfunction
Fatigue
Angina:
    Infrequent
        Due to
            Decreased perfusion: Low diastolic BP
            Increased demand
            Associated CAD
    Nocturnal angina:
        An unusual form of angina in patients with AR with normal coronary arteries
            Occurs in paroxysms
            Usually at night
Palpitations:
    Usually due to forceful LV contraction
    Rarely due to arrhythmias (common in late stage of disease; both ventricular and atrial arrhythmias)

Dizziness: Uncommon

Syncope is **non** existent (compare with AS)

Rapid progression of Dyspnea in AR: Causes
Recurrence of rheumatic activity
Infective endocarditis
Retroversion of aortic cusp
Aortic dissection
Onset of systemic hypertension
Associated CAD

Chronic AR: Signs

Peripheral signs
Present in severe AR in **absence** of CCF

de Musset's sign:	To and fro motion of head synchronous with cardiac cycle
Corrigan's sign:	Visual pulsations of supraclavicular or carotid arteries.
Water-hammer pulse:	High amplitude and abruptly collapsing pulse.
Hill's sign:	Popliteal cuff blood pressure exceeding brachial cuff blood pressure by 20-40 mm Hg: indicates mild AR 40-60 mm Hg: indicates moderate AR > 60 mm Hg: indicates severe AR
Landolfi's sign:	Change in size of pupil synchronous with cardiac cycle
Muller's sign:	Pulsations of uvula
Rosenbach's sign:	Pulsation of liver
Gerhardt's sign:	Pulsation of spleen
Quincke's pulse:	Alternate paling and flushing of lightly compressed skin (nail bed, mucous membrane of mouth)

Pistol-shot femorals:	Booming sound synchronous with systole heard over femoral arteries
Traube's sign:	Double pistol-shot sounds; both systolic and diastolic
Duroziez's sign:	Systolic and diastolic bruits heard over the femoral artery if compressed proximal or distal to the stethoscope respectively (diastolic bruit is the most specific sign)

Arterial pulse

Bisferians pulse
    Hallmark of AR
    Present only in more than moderate AR or AR with AS
        (with predominant AR)
Water-hammer pulse

Blood pressure

*Completely normal blood pressure with clinically normal LV
    function excludes more than moderate AR
With progressive AR, the systolic BP increases and diastolic BP
    falls. But it is unusual for SBP to rise more than 160 mm Hg
    in absence of systemic hypertension.
Degree of decrease in DBP is a better marker of severity of AR
    rather than increase in SBP
DBP: Muffling of Korotkoff sounds is better marker of actual
    DBP; it corresponds to LVEDP and DBP cannot be less than
    maximum LVEDP
        Less than 40 mm Hg almost always indicates free,
            severe AR
        DBP > 60 mm Hg in absence of LV dysfunction or
            systemic hypertension almost rules out severe
            isolated AR.

Pulse pressure more than 50 % of SBP is an unreliable marker of severe AR

Diagnosis of concomitant Hypertension in AR
High Systolic blood pressure can be diagnosed only if end organ damage is present
High Diastolic BP: if it more than 60 mm Hg in presence of signs of free severe AR

Apex beat

Hyperdynamic
Down and out apex beat (E/O LV enlargement) is s/o significant AR
Sustained apex beat in late stage of AR with LV dysfunction results due to increase in LVESV

AR: Auscultation
Auscultation: Sounds

S1: Usually Normal;
    Soft S1:
        Associated with prolong PR interval
        Chronic severe AR with LV dysfunction (High LVEDP resulting in premature closure of MV)
    S2:
        Diminished A2 (**AR due to Aortic Valve Disease**)
        Rheumatic AR
        AS with AR
        Infective endocarditis
        Loud A2 in AR (**AR due to Aortic Root Disease**)
        Syphilis ('Tambour' in quality)
        Marfan's syndrome
        Annuloectasia of Aortic root (Takayasu's aortitis)
        Functional AR due to severe systemic hypertension

Rheumatoid arthritis

Reiter's syndrome

Aortic dissection

Loud A2 with aortic valve disease

(Mechanism of AR in these cases: Prolapse of leaflets)

VSD with AR

TOF with AR

S2 Split:

Closely split or single

Reverse split is uncommon unless associated with LBBB
(compare with AS)

S3:

Present in chronic severe AR

Associated with peripheral signs of AR and high
LVEDV

More commonly present with

LV dysfunction,

Associated MR

* S3 is more common in acute AR (loud S3!) than in
chronic AR

S4:

Presence indicates raised LVEDP in severe AR

Presence indicates severe AR

* S3 and S4 are overall uncommon findings in AR (Dalen and
Alpert)

EC:

Aortic EC may be present; more common with mild
disease

May be due to valve or dilated aortic root

Abrupt distention of aorta due to increased stroke volume causes EC

Disappears with LVF

Auscultation: Murmurs

Three different murmurs can occur

1. EDM: Length is proportional to the severity of AR

High pitched and blowing (high frequency)
Site: Base of the heart;
     2nd RICS or 3rd LICS
     Loudest in 3rd LICS in Rheumatic AR
     3rd RICS if AR is due to dilated Aortic root
     Rarely in elderly patient or patient with chest deformity the murmur is best heard at apex or in left axilla (Cole Cecil murmur)
Decrescendo
     Audible till 'late' diastole in severe AR; duration decreases with onset of CCF
Rarely associated with thrill (i.e., rarely > grade 4)
Increase with sitting position, leaning forward with breath held in expiration
Increase with isometric sustained handgrip, squatting and vasopressors

2. ESM: Systolic flow murmur across AV:

Flow murmur; may not indicate coexisting AS
Usually peaks in first half of systole
May be associated with systolic thrill even in absence of AS

3 Austin Flint murmur:

MDM / presystolic murmur at apex (Similar to MS murmur)

Only with severe AR

Peripheral signs of AR are always present

More common in non rheumatic AR

* Disappearance of preexisting presystolic Austin Flint murmur in AR suggest aggravation of AR or onset of LV failure (Premature closure of MV due to raised LVEDP

Mechanisms: Different proposed explanations are

a. Jet of AR falling on AML preventing adequate opening and causing turbulence to flow across mitral valve in diastole (relative mitral stenosis)

b. Diastolic MR due to raised LVEDP

c. Radiation of low pitched vibrations of AR murmur at apex

d. Flutter of AML

e. Turbulence generated by mixing of antegrade mitral flow and retrograde AR flow (Laniado et al)

Differentiation of MDM of MS from Austin Flint murmur

Features favoring MS:

Loud S1

OS is diagnostic

Diastolic thrill: Diagnostic

LVS3 never occurs in pure MS

Signs of PH

Amyl nitrate increases the murmur

Absence of peripheral signs of AR (in pure MS)

Significant AR with short or no murmur

Acute AR

AR with LV failure

Tachycardia

Hypotension
Vasodilators
Pregnancy

Clinical criteria of Severe AR

- Marked peripheral signs: Bisferiens pulse; Hill's sign > 60 mm Hg
- SBP > 160 ; DBP < 40 ; Pulse Pressure > 50 % of SBP
    Especially with multivalvular involvement
- Hyperdynamic, laterally displaced apical impulse
- EDM: Lasting > 2/3 rd of diastole
- Presence of thrill
- Austin Flint Murmur

Severe AR: Acute Vs Chronic
- Acute
    Absence of
    - CE
    - Peripheral signs
    - Systolic thrill (due to increase in flow)
    Presence of
    - Very severe symptoms
    - Tachycardia
    - S3
    - EDM and diastolic thrill
    - Austin Flint murmur

Clinical Course

Mild Regurgitation is compatible with normal lifestyle
    Asymptomatic
    Only risk is of endocarditis
    Treat with diuretics and vasodilators

Moderate – Severe

> Symptoms appear
>> Dyspnea on exertion or when lying flat
>> Fatigue

Chronic Aortic Regurgitation

> Better tolerated than Aortic Stenosis if compensatory mechanisms occur
> Condition unlikely to improve in the long term
> Surgery should be performed before LV dysfunction occurs

Acute Aortic Regurgitation requires emergency surgery

Investigations

1. **ECG:**

   Following points reflect presence of significant AR:

   > Evidence of LV Hypertrophy
   > Diastolic overload: qR (tall R) with upright T wave in lateral
   >   precordial leads
   > Left axis deviation
   > Conduction defects
   >   Prolong PR interval
   >   Mobitz type I block
   >   LBBB
   >   Less common in rheumatic AR

2. **CXR**

   > LV enlargement: Advance disease: "Boot shaped" heart
   >   No e/o CE till moderate degree of AR
   > Dilation of the ascending Aorta
   > Calcification of AV

3. Echocardiographic assessment of AR

Indispensable tool for evaluation of AR

M Mode features:

Accurately measures
LV internal Diameter in Systole (LVIDS)
LV internal Diameter in Diastole (LVIDD)
Fractional shortening (FS)
LV hypertrophy

Specific features
Chronic AR
Coarse flutter of anterior mitral leaflet (AML) and occasionally of posterior mitral leaflet (PML) in diastole (Not seen if there is associated MS)

Diastolic non coaptation of aortic valve (AV) leaflets

LV volume overload (LVVO)

Acute AR
Premature opening of AV and premature closure of mitral valve (MV)

2 – D Echo:

Establishes the mechanism of AR (e.g., leaflet disease vs. aortic root dilatation)

Features of AR
LVVO
PSAX view:

No. of cusps, incomplete closure of leaflets (> 2 mm),
Vegetation, Root dilatation, Dissection etc
Reverse doming of AML (Bent knee appearance)

PLAX view:
Diastolic flutter of MV leaflet (AML)
Prolapse of leaflet

Doppler Study

Continuous Wave (CW) Doppler

Views: A5C and A2C

Assessment of severity:
1. Pressure half time (PHT) of AR jet
2. Deceleration slope of AR jet
3. Spectral strength of AR jet

1. PHT method:
Amount of time required for the peak diastolic gradient to reduce by 50 % of its peak value. The steeper the slope, lesser the PHT and severe the AR.

PHT > 400 msec: Mild AR
PHT < 200 msec;   Severe AR

2. Deceleration Slope of AR:
Steeper the slope, more severe the AR

Limitation of these 2 methods:

Influenced by
LV compliance
Systemic hypertension,

High systemic vascular resistance,
Associated valvular lesions

3. **Spectral strength of AR jet**:

Not as good as the previous two methods.

Grade 1 +: Faint spectral tracing stains sufficient for detection but complete tracing not seen

Grade 2 +: Complete spectral tracing can just be seen

Grade 3 +: Distinct spectral tracing is seen but the echo density is less than antegrade flow.

Grade 4 +: Echo dense spectral tracing more than the antegrade flow.

Pulse wave (PW) Doppler

The severity of AR is assessed by mapping the depth of the diastolic flow signal of AR extending from base of aortic leaflet into the LV cavity, seen in A5C view.

Grade ! +: Jet extends just beneath the aortic leaflets

Grade 2 +: Jet extends to the tip of mitral leaflets

Grade 3 +: Jet extends to the level of papillary muscles

Grade 4 +: Jet extends beyond papillary muscles

Limitations:
Difficult to assess eccentric jets of AR
Good echo view is necessary to obtain a clear signal
May overestimate the severity in compliant LV

Underestimates the severity in acute AR or in low output states

Color Doppler

Modality of choice for assessment of severity of AR

Assessment of severity of AR by color Doppler:

Length of AR jet
Ratio of AR jet diameter to LVOT diameter
Ratio of AR jet area to LVOT area
Diastolic flow reversal in Aorta
Others

1. Length of AR jet:
Easy but may not be accurate
Gradation similar to Pulse Doppler method

Grade ! +: Jet extends just beneath the aortic leaflets
Grade 2 +: Jet extends to the tip of mitral leaflets
Grade 3 +: Jet extends to the level of papillary muscles
Grade 4 +: Jet extends beyond papillary muscles

Limitations:
Influenced by color gain settings, LV compliance, LVEDP and presence of multivalvular disease.
Underestimates severity of acute AR.

2. Ratio of AR jet diameter to LVOT diameter

Very useful and easily reproducible method
PLAX view

Obtain a good view of AR jet at its origin and measure the diameter at the two ends of AR jet and LVOT diameter at the level of aortic leaflet attachment.

An absolute value of more than 12 mm (AR jet diameter) indicates severe AR

Grading of AR by the ratio of AR jet diameter to LVOT diameter

Grade 1:   Less than 25 %
Grade 2:   25 – 45 %
Grade 3:   45- 65 %
Grade 4:   More than 65 %

3. Ratio of AR jet area to LVOT area

Similar to above method but the PSAX view is used to measure area as the AR jet may not be exactly circular.

Grading of AR by the ratio of AR jet area to LVOT area

Grade 1:   Less than 25 %
Grade 2:   25 – 45 %
Grade 3:   45- 65 %
Grade 4:   More than 65 %

4. Diastolic flow reversal in Aorta

Useful method to differentiate between mild and severe AR

Suprastenal view is used

A diastolic flow reversal is seen in AR (due to backflow into LV cavity). A pandiastolic flow reversal rules our mild AR and denotes an AR of at least moderately severe AR (More than grade 3). An end diastolic flow velocity of more than 0.2 m/s suggest severe AR.

Ratio of diastolic to systolic flow > 60 % indicates at least grade 3 AR

5. Others:

a. Product of area of AR jet at its origin and the velocity time integral (VTI) of AR

AR jet area X VTI AR or
0.75 X Jet diameter at origin X VTI AR
    More than 81 suggest severe AR

b. Vena Contracta
    Good method but still not validated
    12 mm indicates severe AR

c. Quantitative measurement:

(i) **Regurgitant volume (RV)**

RV = Volume retuning to LV during each beat due to regurgitation

Actual Forward SV = Total SV of AV – RV
Therefore,
RV = Total SV of AR – Actual Forward SV

Total SV of AR = LVOT area X VTI LVOT

Actual Forward SV: Measured at Mitral (MV) or Pulmonary valve (PV) as that value reflects the actual forward stroke volume.

Actual forward SV of AV = SV of MV / PV
= MV area / RVOT area X VTI MV / RVOT
Therefore,
RV = SV of AV – SV of MV / PV

RV more than 60 ml indicates severe AR

(ii) **Regurgitant fraction (RF)**

RF = Regurgitant volume / Total Stroke volume X 100

= (SV at AV – SV at MV) / Total SV AV X 100

Grading of AR by RF

Grade 1:	Less than 20 %
Grade 2:	20 – 30 %
Grade 3:	30- 50 %
Grade 4:	More than 50 %

Limitations:
Not applicable in mixed AV disease and multivalvular disease
Difficult, time consuming and needs accuracy in measurements

(iii) **Effective regurgitant orifice (ERO)**

Accurate
An ERO more than 30 mm^2 indicates severe AR

Summary of Echo-Doppler features of Chronic Severe AR

LVID:
  Diastole > 70 mm (38 mm / m²)
  Systole > 50 mm (26 mm / m²)
AR jet diameter / LVOT diameter > 65 %
AR jet area / LVOT area > 65 %
AR jet diameter > 12 mm
RV > 60 ml
RF > 50 %
ERO > 30 mm²
Pandiastolic flow reversal in descending aorta
PHT of AR jet < 200 msec

Echo – Doppler feature of Acute Severe AR

Premature closure of MV (Raised LVEDP)
Premature opening of AV
Early or late diastolic MR
Mitral flow:
  Increased mitral E velocity
  Small or absent A velocity
  Increased E/A ratio
  Shortened deceleration time of MV inflow < 150 msec

4. Cardiac Catheterization

Estimation of severity of AR by aortic root angiography

Degree of regurgitation	Findings
1 + (Trivial)	Reflux of contrast into LV outflow tract during early diastole

2 + (mild)	Reflux of contrast into LV outflow tract during early diastole and present till onset of systole
3 + (moderate)	Contrast fills entire LV including apex and with increasing opacification during successive cycles
4 + (severe)	Contrast fills entire LV chamber during first diastole. It frequently remain visible in LV for 10-15 secs.

Natural History

Salient points

- Latent phase of AR, like AS, may last decades
- Decompensation starts when
    - LV systolic function begins to fail
    - Progressive LV dilatation occurs
    - Spherical geometry develops
- Initially these compensatory mechanisms are reversible
- LV systolic function and ESD are the most important predictors of postoperative survival and LV function
- In asymptomatic patients with severe AR and normal LV systolic function, progression is slow†
    - 4.3% / yr develop symptoms of LV systolic dysfunction
    - 1.3% / yr progress to LV dysfunction without symptoms

† pooled data from 7 series. 490 pts with mean follow-up of 6.4 yrs

Severe AR: Natural History

- Rapaport
    - Survival rate after diagnosis
        - 5 yr: 75 %
        - 10 yr: 50 %

- Symptoms vs. asymptomatic patients
    - Asymtomatic patients
        - Mild to moderate AR: 10 yr survival is 90 %
        - Moderate to severe AR: 10 yr survival is 50 % (75 % at 5 yrs)
    - Symptoms
        - Angina: Mean survival 4 yrs
        - CHF: Mean survival 2 yrs
        - NYHA class III / IV on medical treatment: 5 % survival at 10 yrs.

- Bonow and Ebstein et al (Circ 1991) Natural History of Asymptomatic chronic Severe AR with normal LV function
    - N = 108
    - Diagnosed by cardiac angiography
    - LVEF > 45 %
    - F/U: Mean 8 yrs (2 –16 yrs)
    - F/U by Echo or radionuclide angiography
        - Asymptomatic with normal LV function: 75 %
        - Asymptomatic with decreased LV function: 4 %
        - Required AVR: 19 %
        - Death: 2 %
    - Average attrition rate: 5 % per yr

- Bonow and Ebstein et al: Risk Stratification in chronic severe AR

Variable	Value	Likelihood of death/ symptoms / LV dysfunction
LVIDS	> 50 mm	19 % / yr
	40 –49 mm	6 % / yr
	< 40 mm	0 % / yr

LVIDD	$\geq$ 70 mm	10 % / yr
	< 70 mm	2 % / yr
Change in LVEF	Decrease by > 5 %	12 % / yr
(in response to	Decrease by 0 – 5 %	4 % / yr
Exercise)		
	Increase	1 % / yr

Bonow and Ebstein et al: Indication for AVR based on their study
- Symptomatic severe AR
- Asymptomatic severe AR if
    - Development of LV systolic dysfunction at rest
    - Development of marked LV dilatation
        - LVIDD $\geq$ 80 mm
        - LVIDS $\geq$ 55 mm
        - LVEDV index > 200 ml/m2

Natural History of Chronic Aortic Regurgitation

Asymptomatic patients with normal LV systolic Function
    Progression to symptoms and LV dysfunction < 6 % / yr
    Progression to asymptomatic LV dysfunction <3.5 %/ yr
    Sudden Death <0.2%/yr
Asymptomatic patients with LV systolic dysfunction
    Progression to Cardiac Symptoms >25 % / yr
Symptomatic Patients
    Mortality Rate 10 % / yr

Borer et al (Circ 1998):

Hypothesis: Objective noninvasive measures of LV size and performance and, specifically, of load-adjusted variables, assessed at rest and during exercise, could predict the development of currently accepted indications for operation for AR.

Prediction of indication for valve replacement among asymptomatic or minimally symptomatic patients.

With chronic AR and normal LV performance
- Δ LVEF - Δ ESS index was strongest indicator of progression to any end point or to SCD. Unadjusted Δ LVEF was almost as efficient
- The population tercile at highest risk by ΔLVEF-ΔESS progressed to end points at a rate of 13.3%/y, and the lowest-risk tercile progressed at 1.8%/y.
- Δ LVEF - Δ ESS index:
  - Highest risk: > -17 %
  - Lowest risk: < - 11%

Where,

Δ LVEF: change (Δ) in LV EF from rest to exercise

Δ ESS: change (Δ) in ESS from rest to exercise

Greves et al:
Patients operated for AR had a low 5 yr cardiac mortality if resting LVEF > 50 % regardless of severity of symptoms

Spagnulo et al (Circ 1971; 44; 368-80)
Cardiomegaly on CXR
LVH on ECG
SBP > 140 mm Hg
DBP < 40 mm hg

- Presence of all these predict 87 % chance of becoming symptomatic or dying at 6 yrs

AR: Management

Options:
  Medical Therapy
  Interventions

Medical Therapy

  No specific therapy to prevent disease progression in chronic AR

  Systemic DBP if present should be treated because it increases regurgitant flow. Vasodilators like long acting nifedipine or ACE inhibitors are preferred. However, definite recommendations regarding the indications for long acting nifedipine or ACE inhibitors are not possible as trials have not consistently shown benefits of these drugs in reducing development of symptoms or LV dysfunction.

Vasodilator Therapy in AR

- Expected to decrease afterload, increase stroke volume and decrease regurgitant volume
- Hemodynamic benefit shown with hydralazine and nifedipine, less consistent results with ACE inhibitors

- Improvement in clinical outcomes in trial of LA (long acting) nifedipine vs. digoxin
  - Need for AVR in 143 pts followed for 6 yrs
  - LA Nifedipine Vs. Digoxin: 15% vs 34%
    - Hence vasodilator therapy was better
- Dose titrated to achieve decrease in SBP, not normalization

Medical Therapy: Recommendations

Class I

Vasodilator therapy is indicated for chronic therapy in patients with severe AR who have symptoms or LV dysfunction when surgery is not recommended because of additional cardiac or noncardiac factors. *(Level of Evidence: B)*

Class IIa

Vasodilator therapy is reasonable for short-term therapy to improve the hemodynamic profile of patients with severe heart failure symptoms and severe LV dysfunction before proceeding with AVR. *(Level of Evidence: C)*

Class IIb

Vasodilator therapy may be considered for long-term therapy in asymptomatic patients with severe AR who have LV dilatation but normal systolic function. *(Level of Evidence: B)*

Class III
1. Vasodilator therapy is not indicated for long-term therapy in asymptomatic patients with mild to moderate AR and normal LV systolic function. *(Level of Evidence: B)*
2. Vasodilator therapy is not indicated for long-term therapy in asymptomatic patients with LV systolic dysfunction who are otherwise candidates for AVR. *(Level of Evidence: C)*

3. Vasodilator therapy is not indicated for long-term therapy in symptomatic patients with either normal LV function or mild to moderate LV systolic dysfunction who are otherwise candidates for AVR. *(Level of Evidence: C)*

AR: Interventions

AV Replacement or Repair

Recommendations for AVR

Indications for Aortic Valve Replacement or Aortic Valve Repair

Class I

1. AVR is indicated for symptomatic patients with severe AR irrespective of LV systolic function. *(Level of Evidence: B)*
2. AVR is indicated for asymptomatic patients with chronic severe AR and LV systolic dysfunction (ejection fraction 0.50 or less) at rest. *(Level of Evidence: B)*
3. AVR is indicated for patients with chronic severe AR while undergoing CABG or surgery on the aorta or other heart valves. *(Level of Evidence: C)*

Class IIa

AVR is reasonable for asymptomatic patients with severe AR with normal LV systolic function (ejection fraction greater than 0.50) but with severe LV dilatation (end-diastolic dimension greater than 75 mm or end-systolic dimension greater than 55 mm).* *(Level of Evidence: B)*

Class IIb

1. AVR may be considered in patients with moderate AR while undergoing surgery on the ascending aorta. *(Level of Evidence: C)*

2. AVR may be considered in patients with moderate AR while undergoing CABG. *(Level of Evidence: C)*
3. AVR may be considered for asymptomatic patients with severe AR and normal LV systolic function at rest (ejection fraction greater than 0.50) when the degree of LV dilatation exceeds an end-diastolic dimension of 70 mm or end-systolic dimension of 50 mm, when there is evidence of progressive LV dilatation, declining exercise tolerance, or abnormal hemodynamic responses to exercise.* *(Level of Evidence: C)*

Class III

AVR is not indicated for asymptomatic patients with mild, moderate, or severe AR and normal LV systolic function at rest (ejection fraction greater than 0.50) when degree of dilatation is not moderate or severe (end-diastolic dimension less than 70 mm, end-systolic dimension less than 50 mm).* *(Level of Evidence: B)*

Consider lower threshold values for patients of small stature of either gender.

Summary:

Severe AR: Indication for Sx

- Symptomatic severe AR
- Acute AR
- Infective Endocarditis Of AV
- Asymptomatic severe AR if
    E/O LV dysfunction at rest
    - LVEF < 50%   FS < 27 %

    With normal LV function if
- LVIDD   > 70 mm (38 mm/m2)
- LVIDS   > 50 mm (26 mm/m2)

- LVESVI   > 60 ml/m2
- LVEDVI   > 180 ml/m2
- (SBP X LV End diastolic radius) /
  Wall thickness   > 600
- LV end diastolic radius /
  Wall thickness   > 3.8
- LVSP / LVESV   < 1.72 mm Hg/ml/m2

                           (> 1.72 very strong predictor of
  good outcome after surgery)

  Where

       LVSP: LV systolic pressure

       LVESV: LV end systolic volume

- Δ LVEF - Δ ESS index: - 17 % (Increase risk of poor outcome)
- ESS / ESVI : Preload independent and partial afterload independent

       Normal > 4.9; In AR always < 4.9

       If > 2.9: Ratio normalizes post operatively in nearly all

       If < 2.9: Ratio will not normalize and patient will have LV dysfunction post operatively

- Progressive cardiomegaly on CXR
- Progressive LVH on ECG

AVR: Survival after Surgery

1. Depends on LVEF before operation

LVEF preoperatively	5 Yr survival
> 50 %	90 – 100 %
< 50 %	69 %

2. Tajk and Klodes et al: On basis of symptom class of patients

NYHA Class I / II
    i.   Operative mortality   1 – 2 %
    ii.   10 yr survival   78 +/- 4 %

NYHA Class III / IV
    iii.   Operative mortality   7 – 8 %
    iv.   10 yr survival   45 + / - 5 %

AVR: Operative risk

Increased risk for operative mortality
(J Card Surg 1987 Dec 2 (4); 435 -452)
- Associated AS
- NYHA class III / IV
- Age > 65 yrs
- CTR > 65 %
- EF < 45 %
- CI < 2.2 L/min/m2
- ESD > 55 mm
- ESVI > 200 ml/m2
- LV systolic pressure / LVESV < 1.72

AVR with Root Replacement (Bentall's procedure)
If significant aortic root enlargement is present (> 5 cm diameter)
AVR is performed as valve conduit.

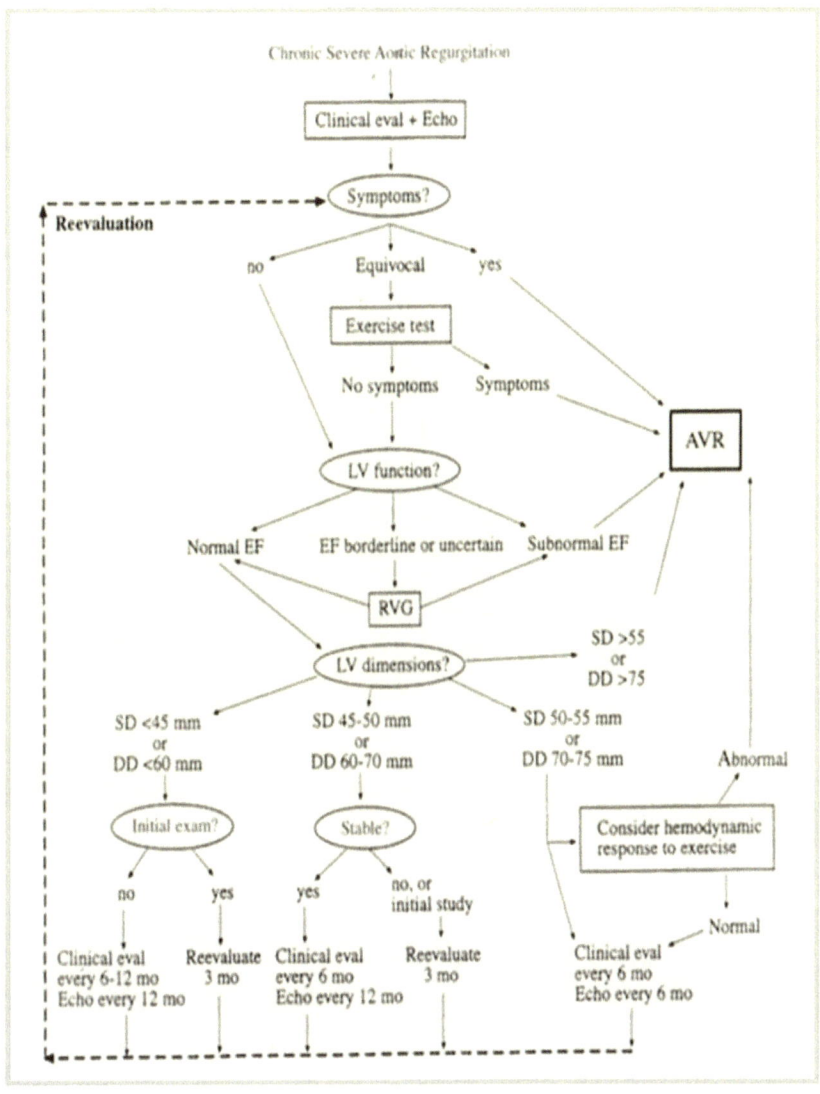

Based on ACC / AHA 2006 guidelines for the management of patients with valvular heart disease.

Suggested Reading

1. Chapter 52: Acquired Aortic Valve Disease. *Surgery of the Chest* (Sabiston and Spencer), 5th ed., 1566-96.

2. Chapter 12: Aortic Valve Disease. *Cardiac Surgery* (Kirklin and Barratt-Boyes), 2nd ed., 491-572.

3. Chapter 120: Aortic Valve Disease and Hypertrophic Cardiomyopathies. *Glenn's Thoracic and Cardiovascular Surgery* (Baue, Geha, Hammond, Laks, and Naunheim), 6th ed., 1981-2004.

4. Rapaport E: Calculation of valve areas. Eur Heart J 1985; 6 (suppl C): 21.

5. Ohlsson J, Wranne B: Noninvasive assessment of valve area in patients with aortic stenosis. J Am Coll Cardiol 1986; 7: 501.

6. Lombard JT, Selzer A: Valvular aortic stenosis: a clinical and hemo-dynamic profile of patients. Ann Intern Med 1987; 106: 292.

7. Goldschlager N, Pfeifer J, Cohn K, Popper R, Selzer A: The natural history of aortic regurgitation: a clinical and hemodynamic study. Am J Med 1973; 54: 577.

8. Bonow RO, Rosing DR, McIntosh CL, et al: The natural history of asymptomatic patients with aortic regurgitation and normal left ventricular function. Circulation 1983; 68: 509.

9. Otto CM. Valvular aortic stenosis: Disease severity and timing of intervention. J Am Coll Cardiol. 2006, 47: 2141-2151.

10. Enriquez-Sarano M, Tajik AJ. Aortic regurgitation. N Engl J Med. 2004, 351: 1539-1546.

11. Bekeredjian R, Grayburn PA. Valvular heart disease: Aortic regurgitation. Circulation. 2005, 112: 125-134.

12. Scognamiglio R, Rahimtoola SH, Fasoli G, et al: Nifedipine in asymptomatic patients with severe aortic regurgitation and normal left ventricular function. N Engl J Med. 1994, 331: 689-694.

13. American College of Cardiology; American Heart Association Task Force on Practice Guidelines (Writing Committee to revise the 1998 guidelines for the management of patients with valvular heart disease); Society of Cardiovascular Anesthesiologists; Bonow RO, Carabello BA, Chatterjee K, et al: ACC/AHA 2006 guidelines for the management of patients with valvular heart disease. J Am Coll Cardiol. 2006, 48: e1-e148.

14. Chapter 66: Valvular Heart Disease. Braunwald's Heart Disease(Elsevier), 9th ed., 1468-1539.

15. Chapters 6: Aortic Stenosis. Valvular Heart Disease. Edited by Dalen and Alpert (Little, brown and company). 2th ed., 197-282

16. Chapters 7: Chronic Aortic Regurgitation. Valvular Heart Disease. Edited by Dalen and Alpert (Little, brown and company). 2th ed., 283-318

17. Chapters 8: Acute Aortic insufficiency. Valvular Heart Disease. Edited by Dalen and Alpert (Little, brown and company). 2th ed., 319-352

Abbreviations

ACE:	Angiotensin converting enzyme
A2:	Aortic component of second heart sound
A2C:	Apical two chamber
A4C:	Apical four chamber
A5C:	Apical five chamber
AF:	Atrial Fibrillation
AI:	Aortic insufficiency / Aortic incompetence
AML:	Anterior mitral leaflet
AR:	Aortic Regurgitation
AS:	Aortic Stenosis
AV:	Aortic Valve
AVG:	Aortic valve gradient
AVA:	Aortic Valve Area
AVR:	Aortiv valve replacement
AV:	Aortic Valve
AV block:	Atrio-ventricular block
AV dissociation:	Atrio-ventricular dissociation
BAV:	Balloon aortic valvotomy
BP:	Blood pressure
CI:	Cardiac index
CABG:	Coronary artery bypass graft surgery
CAD:	Coronary artery disease
CCF:	Congestive cardiac failure
CE:	Cardiac enlargement
CHF:	Congestive heart failure
CT:	Computed tomography
CTR:	Cardio thoracic ratio
CXR:	Chest X-ray

DBP:	Diastolic Blood pressure
D/D:	Differential diagnosis
DSE:	Dobutamine stress test
EC:	Ejection click
ECG:	Electrocardiogram
EDM:	Early diastolic murmur
EF:	Ejection fraction
EI:	Eccentricity index
E/O:	Evidence of
ERO:	Effective regurgitant orifice
ESD:	End systolic diameter
ESM:	Ejection systolic murmur
ESS:	End systolic stress
ESV:	End systolic volume
ESVI:	End systolic volume index
F/U:	Follow up
Fr:	French
FS:	Fractional shortening
GI:	Gastrointestinal
HOCM:	Hypertrophic obstructive cardiomyopathy
ICS:	Intercostal space
IE:	Infective endocarditis
IHJ:	Indian Heart Journal
IV:	Intra-venous
IVS:	Inter ventricular septum
LA:	Left atrium
LAE:	Left atrial enlargement
LAP:	Left atrial pressure
LBBB:	Left bundle branch block

LCX:	Left circumflex
LICS:	Left intercostal space
LV:	Left ventricle
LVEF:	Left ventricular ejection fraction
LVEDP:	Left ventricular end diastolic pressure
LVEDV:	Left ventricular end diastolic volume
LVEDVI:	Left ventricular end diastolic volume index
LVESV:	Left ventricular end systolic volume
LVESVI:	Left ventricular end systolic volume index
LVF:	Left ventricular failure
LVH:	Left ventricular hypertrophy
LVID:	LV internal Diameter
LVIDS:	LV internal Diameter in Systole
LVIDD:	LV internal Diameter in Diastole
LVSP:	Left ventricular systolic pressure
LVOT:	Left ventricle outflow tract
LVOTO:	Left ventricle outflow tract obstruction
LVVO:	Left ventricular volume overload
MR:	Mitral Regurgitation
MS:	Mitral stenosis
MV:	Mitral Valve
MDM:	Mid diastolic murmur
MVD:	Mitral Valve disease
NYHA:	New York Heart Association
OS:	Opening snap
P2:	Pulmonary component of second heart sound
PAH:	Pulmonary arterial hypertension
PAWP:	Pulmonary artery wedge pressure
PH:	Pulmonary hypertension
PHT:	Pressure half time
PLAX:	Parasternal long axis

PML:	Posterior mitral leaflet
PND:	Paroxysmal nocturnal dyspnea
PSAX:	Parasternal short axis
PV:	Pulmonary valve
RA:	Right atrium
RAP:	Right atrial pressure
RF:	Regurgitant fraction
RHD:	Rheumatic heart disease
RICS:	Right intercostal space
RSOV:	Ruptured sinus of Valsalva
RV:	Right ventricle
RV:	Regurgitant volume
RVEDP:	Right ventricular end diastolic pressure
RVOT:	Right ventricle outflow tract
RVSP:	Right ventricular systolic pressure
Rx:	Treatment
S1:	First heart sound
S2:	Second heart sound
S3:	Third heart sound
S4:	Third heart sound
SAM:	Systolic anterior motion
SBP:	Systolic Blood pressure
SCD:	Sudden cardiac death
SLE:	Systemic lupus erythematous
SM:	Systolic murmur
STS:	Society of Thoracic Surgeons
SV:	Stroke volume
TAVI:	Trans-catheter aortic valve implantation
TEE:	Trans esophageal echocardiography
TMT:	Treadmill Test
TOF:	Tetralogy Of Fallot
TTE:	Trans thoracic echocardiography

TR:	Tricuspid Regurgitation
TS:	Tricuspid stenosis
TV:	Tricuspid valve
VACA:	Valvuloplasty and Angioplasty in Congenital Anomalies
VSD:	Ventricular septal defect
VTI:	Velocity time integral

About the Author

The author is an interventional cardiologist. He has completed his cardiology training from prestigious G S Seth Medical czollege and KEM Hospital, Mumbai, India. He has worked as cardiology fellow in Galsgow Royal Infirmary, Glasgow for 1 year. After completion of fellowship he has been practicing cardiology in Gujarat, India for ten years. He has vast experience in Coronary as well as Rheumatic heart disease (RHD). RHD is still quite common in India and is a major cause of admission in hospitals. The author has rich experience of balloon valvuloplasties. His experience in dealing with valvular heart disease gives him an edge in writing a detailed book about aortic valve disease. He has also published "A Handbook of Rheumatic Fever" with Authorhouse. Apart from this handbook he has been a co-author of a book called "Patel's Atlas on Transradial Interventions: The basics".

The author has compiled the details about the aortic valve disease in great details and is sure the handbook will be very useful to students as well as practitioners.

www.ingramcontent.com/pod-product-compliance
Lightning Source LLC
Chambersburg PA
CBHW031237280526
45784CB00004B/1618